Self-System Therapy
for Depression

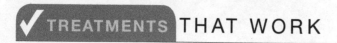

✔TREATMENTS THAT WORK

Self-System Therapy for Depression

CLIENT WORKBOOK

KARI M. EDDINGTON

TIMOTHY J. STRAUMAN

ANGELA Z. VIETH

GREGORY G. KOLDEN

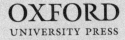

OXFORD
UNIVERSITY PRESS

OXFORD
UNIVERSITY PRESS

Oxford University Press is a department of the University of Oxford. It furthers
the University's objective of excellence in research, scholarship, and education
by publishing worldwide. Oxford is a registered trade mark of Oxford University
Press in the UK and certain other countries.

Published in the United States of America by Oxford University Press
198 Madison Avenue, New York, NY 10016, United States of America.

© Oxford University Press 2018

ISBN 978–0–19–060248–2

9 8 7 6 5 4 3 2 1

Printed by Webcom, Inc., Canada

One of the most difficult problems confronting patients with various disorders and diseases is finding the best help available. Everyone is aware of friends or family who have sought treatment from a seemingly reputable practitioner, only to find out later from another doctor that the original diagnosis was wrong or the treatments recommended were inappropriate or perhaps even harmful. Most patients, or family members, address this problem by reading everything they can about their symptoms, seeking out information on the Internet or aggressively "asking around" to tap knowledge from friends and acquaintances. Governments and health care policymakers are also aware that people in need do not always get the best treatments—something they refer to as *variability in health care practices*.

Now health care systems around the world are attempting to correct this variability by introducing *evidence-based practice*. This simply means that it is in everyone's interest that patients get the most up-to-date and effective care for a particular problem. Health care policymakers have also recognized that it is very useful to give consumers of health care as much information as possible, so that they can make intelligent decisions in a collaborative effort to improve physical health and mental health. This series, Treatments *ThatWork*, is designed to accomplish just that. Only the latest and most effective interventions for particular problems are described in user-friendly language. To be included in this series, each treatment program must pass the highest standards of evidence available, as determined by a scientific advisory board. Thus, when individuals suffering from these problems, or their family members, seek out an expert clinician who is familiar with these interventions and decides that they are appropriate, patients will have confidence they are receiving the best care available. Of course, only your health care professional can decide on the right mix of treatments for you.

This particular program presents the first evidence-based psychological treatment for depression that focuses on correcting problems with self-regulation. Self-regulation involves the process of setting personal goals and being able to reach them—that is, striving to be the kind of person you want to be. Problems with self-regulation, such as when you negatively evaluate yourself and don't reevaluate your goals or behavior, can result in depression. Thus, Self-System Therapy (SST), as outlined in this treatment, targets improving the process of self-regulation, thereby decreasing feelings of self-disappointment and increasing self-satisfaction to relieve depression symptoms. This Workbook, to be used in conjunction with your treatment provider, provides a description of SST in simple terms with helpful worksheets and exercises.

David H. Barlow, Editor-in-Chief,
Treatments *ThatWork*
Boston, MA

Accessing Treatments *ThatWork* Forms and Worksheets Online

All forms and worksheets from books in the TTW series are made available digitally shortly following print publication. You may download, print, save, and digitally complete them as PDF's. To access the forms and worksheets, please visit http://www.oup.com/us/ttw.

Contents

Self-System Therapy
for Depression

CHAPTER 1 ▸ Overview of the Program

What Is Depression?

Depression is among the most common mental health problems in the world. Most people can describe times when have felt down or "blue," but these experiences are often mild and temporary. Anyone who has been diagnosed with depression by a psychologist or medical doctor knows that feeling a little down is nothing compared with the unrelenting sadness and hopelessness of clinical depression. You are not alone. The World Health Organization estimates that 350 million people worldwide suffer from depression. The rate for women is almost double the rate for men.

Your therapist has probably asked you many questions about the problems you have been having and how long you have had them. You might have discussed with your therapist what it means to be diagnosed with depression, including what the differences are between just feeling down and being clinically depressed. The following is a checklist of symptoms that define clinical depression (also called major depressive disorder), and many of them may be familiar to you:

✓ Feeling sad, depressed, or irritable
✓ Loss of interest or pleasure in things that you would normally enjoy if you were not depressed
✓ Change in sleep (i.e., sleeping too much or too little)
✓ Gaining or losing a significant amount of weight
✓ Loss of energy or feeling tired
✓ Difficulties concentrating or making simple decisions

✓ Feelings of worthlessness or guilt
✓ Feeling either fidgety or very slowed down
✓ Thoughts of death or suicide

In clinical depression, at least five of these symptoms (which must include sadness or loss of interest, or both) must be present most of the day almost every day and must cause impairment. In other words, they must interfere with the things you need to do in your daily life such as taking care of yourself or other people, going to work or school, and enjoying social activities or hobbies. Sometimes, there is a fine line between a normal sad mood (e.g., after a relationship ends, when a loved one passes away) and a diagnosis such as major depressive disorder. Only a qualified professional can determine whether your symptoms cross that line.

Depression: The Motivation Thief

Depression robs people of the ability to enjoy the pleasures of life, such as enjoying a favorite meal, going for a walk on a beautiful day, or feeling proud after completing a difficult task. You probably do experience those positive feelings when you are not depressed. Depression dampens positive feelings and can take them away completely. When you know you are not going to enjoy something, it is hard to get motivated to do it. How many times in the past few weeks have thoughts such as the following run through your head?

Why should I go through all the trouble to cook my favorite meal when it won't even taste that great?

Why should I bother picking out something nice to wear if I'll end up feeling terrible about myself anyway?

Or you can fill in the blank for yourself:

Why should I bother with _____*?*

Because many things, such as going for walks or spending time on your appearance, do not feel pleasant or satisfying, you may have simply given up on them. It is completely understandable. There may be other things that you have not given up on, but you feel as if you are not doing them very well—you seem to be spinning your wheels without moving forward. It is hard to stay motivated when it seems that your efforts are not paying off.

As you have been reading this chapter, some things may have come to mind for you—examples of things that depression has stolen from you. Take a few minutes to think about things you have stopped doing since becoming depressed, things that you have enjoyed in the past, when you were not depressed. Think about everyday activities that used to make you feel proud, satisfied, or pleased. After you have had a chance to think about these things, write them down in the blank lines that follow:

What depression has stolen from me:

1. _____

2. _____

3. _____

4. _____

5. _____

6. _____

An Introduction to This Therapy

For most people, depression involves disappointments and frustrations. As you made the list, you may have considered the fact that the person you see yourself as right now is not the person you used to be and not the person you want to be. How can you change that? It is not easy, but that is one of the main goals of this therapy—helping people like you, people struggling with depression, to be more like the person they want to be.

> **Self-regulation is the process of setting and pursuing goals that help you be the person you want to be.**

There are several reasons depression makes it difficult for you to be who you want to be. The symptoms of depression previously listed make it extremely difficult, if not impossible, for you to accomplish the goals and tasks of everyday life. As a result, you end up feeling disappointed in yourself - as if you are constantly failing. With the help of your therapist, you can look closely at how depression has interfered with your life. You will focus especially on how depression has interfered with your ability to achieve the goals that help you be the person you want to be (or the person you think you should be)—a process called *self-regulation*.

What To Expect from This Therapy

Your therapy is divided into the three phases, as described in Table 1.1.

Your therapist's job is to guide you through the phases. She or he will be approaching your treatment in a very collaborative manner. That means you will be working together as a team, and each of you has an important role.

The Therapist's Role

Your therapist has the role of the expert; he or she is very knowledgeable about depression and, specifically, about how problems with self-regulation contribute to and are caused by depression. Your therapist will gather

Table 1.1. Phases of This Therapy

Therapy Phase	What to Expect
Orientation phase	▪ You will learn more about this therapy. ▪ Your therapist will learn more about your struggles. ▪ You will start to reclaim some of what depression has stolen from you.
Exploration phase	▪ You and your therapist will look at how you see yourself and the standards you set for yourself. ▪ You will keep track of your goals in everyday life situations and help your therapist understand how you pursue those goals.
Adaptation phase	▪ Your therapist will help you look at whether your standards are helping you or getting in your way; you will look closely at the ones that are getting in your way. ▪ You will get specific training in how to be more effective in pursuing the goals that are most important to you.

information from you about your current and past experiences. The therapist will help you put all of that information together to figure out what changes will be most helpful in relieving your depression and will work with you to start making those changes.

Your Role

You also have the role of the expert in this process because you are, after all, the one who knows the most about yourself. The more you can help your therapist understand your perspective on things and the struggles you are having day to day, the more your therapist can help you.

Coming to your sessions prepared to talk openly with your therapist is a great first step. Your therapist will frequently ask you to do small assignments between sessions. These assignments usually do not take much time, but it is extremely important that you complete them. They will help your therapist understand your experiences and will help you apply what you are learning to your everyday life. If you feel that the assignments are too difficult or upsetting, you should tell your therapist so that he or she can help make them more manageable.

> Between-session assignments help your therapist understand your experiences and help you learn to apply therapy skills in your day-to-day life, which can help your recovery.

We recommend weekly therapy sessions, which will keep the momentum going during your recovery while allowing enough time between sessions to complete assignments and apply what you are learning.

What to Expect in a Session

Each session in the treatment program has specific goals and tasks. This is a *structured* type of therapy, which means that your therapist has specific plans for what you will be doing in each session. If you have been in therapy or counseling before but it was unstructured, you may be accustomed to meeting with your therapist or counselor and talking about things that are on your mind that day. In a structured therapy such as this one, your therapist is still interested in what is on your mind, but there is a narrower focus. Your therapist is interested in things you have been thinking about that are relevant to the goals of therapy. This narrower focus allows therapy to progress more quickly. Although each therapist has his or her own style, each session in this program will likely include the following elements:

- A check-in on your current mood and symptoms and any urgent problems that have come up since the previous session.
- A review of any assignment that you completed since the previous session; be sure to tell your therapist about any problems you had.
- A discussion of the main topic for the current session, such as learning new information or skills, exploring your experiences with self-regulation, or looking for common themes in your experiences.
- Preparation of a between-session assignment for the upcoming week, which is created by you and your therapist together.

About This Workbook

This workbook contains worksheets that are used throughout the course of treatment. If you flip through the entire workbook, it may seem a bit daunting, but keep in mind that your therapist will be helping you along the way, coaching you on how to use each worksheet, and answering any questions. You may not use all of the worksheets. Your therapist will tailor the treatment to fit your particular needs, and some of the worksheets and exercises may not fit your situation. Your therapist also may use additional worksheets or materials that are not contained in this workbook to tailor the program to your unique situation. This workbook is not intended as a stand-alone self-help book, and it should be used only in the context of individual therapy with a qualified professional.

This treatment program emphasizes collaboration. The most productive sessions are those in which you and your therapist are prepared for the session and are ready to work together. To help with that, you can remember to bring this workbook with you to each session so that you are ready to take a look at a specific section or worksheet. Feel free to write in this book—take notes, highlight important points, dog-ear the pages, and jot down questions—whatever helps you most!

Is This Therapy Right for You?

Your therapist knows whether this therapy is right for you based on the assessment that was done to evaluate your current symptoms and difficulties. Now that you know something about what this treatment program is all about, you can also decide whether it is a good fit.

Earlier, you were asked to write down examples of the pleasurable and satisfying experiences that depression has stolen from you. Was it easy for you to come up with them? We also said that people with depression often struggle with being the person they want to be. Do you struggle with that too? If you answered yes to either of these questions, this therapy can help you.

We also described the structure of the therapy and what is expected of you to get the most out of this program. If you are ready to work collaboratively with your therapist and do some work between sessions on your own, then this therapy is right for you.

The first goal when you begin this program is to learn about self-regulation and how it is related to your problems with depression. Before we get to that, think about how depression has been getting in the way of things in your everyday life. Then think carefully about each of the questions on Worksheet 1: *How Depression Has Affected Me* at the end of this chapter, and write down your answers. Remember that the worksheets in this workbook are being used for your own benefit; do not be concerned about grammar or spelling.

Self-Regulation: Being Who You Want To Be

You may not know it, but all of the things you wrote down in response to the three questions in Worksheet 1 probably involve problems with *self-regulation*. In Chapter 1, we said that self-regulation is the process of setting and pursuing goals that help you be the person you want to be. Everyone self-regulates; it is how we keep ourselves in check and headed in the right direction. For example, if being a person who is friendly is important to you, you can do things to achieve that goal (call it your *friendliness* goal), such as welcoming a new neighbor or making small talk while waiting in line at the grocery store.

When you follow through with those goals, you feel pleased with yourself. When you do not (for example, you do not welcome the new neighbor), you probably feel disappointed, sad, or frustrated with yourself. Every time you see that neighbor in the driveway, it may remind you that you failed at your friendliness goal, and you again feel upset. Even though you want to be a friendly person, you perhaps never thought about that characteristic as being a friendliness *goal*.

Goals are not always things that we state explicitly or write down. Often we do not think of certain characteristics we value (such as being friendly, athletic, or funny) as goals, but in fact they are. We are motivated to have those characteristics, just as we are motivated by more concrete things, such as earning money.

There are many different types of goals. Goals can be very abstract (e.g., "to be a friendly person"), and an abstract goal can mean lots of things to different people. If we want to get more specific, we can think of many ways to define what it means to be friendly, such as "always welcome new neighbors," "approach strangers at parties," or "get to know classmates."

Throughout this program, your therapist will ask about your goals. Try to think about abstract and concrete goals in a broad sense—as things that motivate you to act or to be a certain way.

> The term *goal* is used broadly in this program. Goals can be very specific and concrete or more abstract.

Promotion and Prevention Goals: A Question of Why

Goals are important for emotional well-being. People typically pursue two types of goals, and each type is connected with certain emotional experiences. Because you and your therapist will be talking about these two kinds of goals throughout the course of the treatment program, we offer a quick introduction.

Promotion goals involve trying to make good things happen (i.e., promoting good things). Returning to our friendliness goal, if you said that you wanted to do all of those friendly things because you enjoy meeting new people and getting to know those around you, you have stated a promotion goal.

> Promotion goals involve trying to make something good happen.
>
> Prevention goals involve trying to keep something bad from happening.

Prevention goals involve trying to keep bad things from happening (i.e., preventing bad things). If you said that you wanted to do all of those friendly things because you do not want people to think you are rude or unsociable, you have stated a prevention goal.

As you can see from the friendliness example, the main difference between the two types of goals involves determining *why* you want to act a certain way or do a certain activity. What is the outcome you are aiming for? On the surface, the goals look the same—both involve acting friendly. However, the *whys* are different: because I enjoy getting to know people (promotion) versus not looking like a rude person (prevention). And you may very well want both!

There can be many reasons why people act a certain way. However, even when there are multiple reasons, there is usually one that is most important and overshadows all of the others. Do not worry if that seems confusing; your therapist will be helping you figure out whether your goals fall into the promotion or prevention category as you discuss them together.

Promotion and Prevention Goals: Emotions

Promotion and prevention goals are connected with certain emotional experiences. Starting with prevention goals, think about a recent time when there was a major weather threat in your area (such as a tornado, flood, hurricane, or snowstorm). You probably had many prevention goals, such as protecting yourself, your house, and your loved ones, and you may have taken actions that were consistent with those goals (for example, taking shelter in a safe area). Focusing on prevention goals is wise under those circumstances. After the threat had passed, assuming there was no damage, you were probably feeling relieved and safe. If, however, a tree fell and took out your fence, you probably felt worried and tense. Despite your best efforts, you were not able to prevent an unpleasant thing from happening.

We can contrast this with promotion goals. Think about a time when you took a vacation or went somewhere you really wanted to go (such as to a museum, or to watch a favorite sports team play). You probably had a lot of promotion goals focused on things such as enjoying yourself, being able to sleep in or stay up late, and spending quality time with others. Assuming that the trip or visit was a success, you probably felt a strong sense of pleasure and joy. If things did not go so well (perhaps the game got rained out or your flight was delayed), you probably felt disappointed, frustrated, or sad. Box 2.1 provides examples of promotion goals, and Box 2.2 gives examples of prevention goals.

Box 2.1 Promotion Goals: Making Good Things Happen

Examples:

- Making a nice meal for the pleasure of it
- Going for a walk to energize myself
- Graduating from college so I can have the career I want
- Being an effective parent because I love my child
- Learning a new skill to satisfy my curiosity or interest

Successful progress → feeling **satisfied, happy, proud, pleased**
Failure or lack of progress → feeling **disappointed, frustrated, sad**

Box 2.2 Prevention Goals: Keeping Bad Things from Happening

Examples:

- Making a nice meal because it is my responsibility
- Going for a walk because I want to keep from gaining weight
- Graduating from college so that I do not disappoint my family
- Being an effective parent so that my children are kept safe
- Learning a new skill to keep from becoming obsolete at work

Successful progress → feeling **relieved, relaxed, reassured, secure**
Failure or lack of progress → feeling **anxious, nervous, worried, tense**

What Does All of This Have To Do with Depression?

What happens when we do not focus enough on making good things happen (i.e., promotion goals)? We miss out on opportunities to experience strong, positive emotions, and we tend to feel down and disappointed. What happens if we focus too much on keeping bad things from happening (i.e., prevention goals)? We tend to feel a lot of tension and anxiety.

Both promotion and prevention goals are important, but to feel our best, it is important to have a *balance* between the two. With depression, that balance tends to be off: there are too few promotion goals, and there may be too much of a focus on prevention goals. One of the things you and your therapist will be working on in this program is shifting the balance so that you can increase the experience of positive emotion in your daily life and decrease the negative emotions.

It's important to strike a balance between promotion and prevention

Worksheet 1: How Depression Has Affected Me

What disappointments, frustrations, or failures have you experienced recently?

_____

_____

_____

_____

_____

_____

What goals or responsibilities have you been having difficulty with recently?

_____

_____

_____

_____

_____

_____

_____

What behaviors or personal characteristics have you been feeling upset about recently?

_____

_____

_____

_____

_____

_____

_____

The second goal of the orientation phase is to look at where your particular "style" of self-regulation came from. Style is your tendency to focus on promotion or prevention goals. Perhaps you already know what your tendency is, but most people do not, and your therapist will be helping you figure that out.

Relationships and Your Regulatory Style

One way of uncovering your regulatory style is to look at how your relationships and interactions with other people—important people in your life such as your parents—helped you learn how to self-regulate.

An example is Jessie, who grew up in a household with very strict rules. Her parents enforced those rules at all times; when Jessie violated a rule, her parents were very unhappy, and she was punished. For example, when she was 5 years old, Jessie went to her friend's house across the street without telling her parents. When she later came home, her parents yelled at her and took away her favorite stuffed animal. This was a typical scenario. When Jessie did not act the way her parents expected her to, unpleasant things happened. Over time, Jessie became vigilant about obeying the rules and constantly focused her attention on trying to keep bad things from happening. If you recognize this as a prevention focus, bravo! You are catching on!

Our parents are not the only ones who have expectations about how we should act, and the expectations do not stop after we become adults. Take a moment to think about *who you are* in all of your different life roles. You may be a son, father, employee, volleyball team member, and husband. In each role, you interact with other people who expect you to be a certain way. Maybe your spouse expects you to be affectionate, neat, handy, and sympathetic. Your boss expects you to be reliable, creative, assertive, and organized. All of these expectations have consequences. If you are not the reliable, creative, assertive, organized person your boss expects you to be, you may receive criticism, miss out on opportunities, or even get fired.

You and your therapist will be spending some time in session talking about the important past and present relationships in your life. Your therapist will ask you questions about the expectations and standards that other people have for you. You probably are not used to thinking about these things, and you may find that doing so takes some time, which is okay. The first step is an easy one. You simply need to make a list of all the important people in your life.

Worksheet 2: *Important People in My Life* provides 10 blanks, 5 for current relationships and 5 for past ones. You do not need to fill in all of the blanks. It is fine if you can come up with only a few names. If you have more than 10, you should trim the list down a bit. Try to narrow it down to the people who really had an impact on you, or ones you have spent or currently spend a lot of time with. For example, you might have had an aunt who lived down the street. You saw her at every family gathering but really did not talk to her much, so you could exclude her from your list.

After you have completed your list of important people, you will be asked to provide more information about each one using the next worksheet. Exploring these relationships can help you and your therapist better understand your goals and your ideas about the person you are and the person you are trying to be (or not to be). Think carefully about each of the following questions for each of the relationships you listed in Worksheet 2. To keep it simple, all of the questions are worded in the past tense, but they also apply to current relationships. Use Worksheet 3: *Exploring Important Relationships* to jot down your answers, first for people from your past and then for people from the present.

- What kind of person did you usually **try to be** around this person, or how did you act (e.g., assertive, supportive, patient, affectionate, childish, obedient)?

- What kind of person did **_he or she_** want you to be or not be (e.g., responsible, adventurous, controlling)? What kinds of standards or expectations did this person have for you?
- What happened when you did not act as this person wanted or expected you to act? For example, did the person get angry with you, ignore you, or punish you?

While working on Worksheet 3, you may notice that you act somewhat differently around different people in your life. For example, you may be more spontaneous when you are with your friends than when you are with your family, perhaps because your family members rely on you to be a person who always plans ahead. You may find that sometimes other people's expectations are in conflict with what you want for yourself. For example, you may really want to relax and enjoy a holiday, but your family expects you to do all the planning. Conflicts such as these are common, and this therapy program can help you be more effective in handling them.

In later sections of this workbook, you will be encouraged to think about how other people's expectations of you (i.e., the standards they set for you) come into play as you go about your daily activities at home, at work, in school, and in your social interactions.

Worksheet 2: Important People in My Life

List the names of *individuals who have played an important role in your life* along with the nature of the relationship (e.g., mother, friend). In the left column, list people from your past; they may be people you no longer talk to or see. In the right column, list individuals you currently interact with in your day-to-day life. You do not need to use all of the blanks, and the order of your entries does not matter.

People from your past	People you interact with currently
Name: Relation:	Name: Relation:
Name: Relation:	Name: Relation:
Name: Relation:	Name: Relation:
Name: Relation:	Name: Relation:
Name: Relation:	Name: Relation:

Worksheet 3: Exploring Important Relationships

Use the list of names from Worksheet 2 to fill in the blanks below:

Important people: Relationships from your past			
Name of important person	How you acted around that person or the kind of person you tried to be	Person's expectations of you	Consequences of violating the person's expectations

Important people: Your current relationships

Name of important person	How you act around that person or the kind of person you try to be	Person's expectations of you	Consequences of violating the person's expectations

What You Are Doing

In Chapter 2, we said that depression often involves focusing too little on promotion goals. It is important to set promotion goals and make progress on them because these types of goals provide opportunities for experiencing pleasant feelings. When people achieve promotion goals, they feel a sense of accomplishment and may feel proud, pleased, or happy. The third goal in the orientation phase is to get you started focusing on promotion goals.

Your therapist will start by looking at how you are spending your time each day in a typical week. During this ordinary, run-of-the-mill week, do not try to alter your usual activities; that will come later. For now, your therapist just wants to know what an ordinary week looks like for you. Worksheet 4: *My Daily Activities* has space for you to track 6 days of your activities from the time you get up in the morning until you go to bed at night. You do not need to provide much detail; a few words in each time slot will do (e.g., "Walked the dog," "Ran errands with a friend"). Because your therapist may ask you to complete Worksheet 4 more than once, you should make several blank copies of it for future use.

What You Are Not Doing

After you have provided the therapist with some information about what you are doing day to day, she or he will look at what you are not doing to determine what is missing. Which activities could help you get closer to your goals? Which activities could help you feel a sense of reward, accomplishment, or progress? In Chapter 1, we described depression as a motivation thief because it robs you of satisfaction and pleasure in things that you used to enjoy before you became depressed. Using Worksheet 5: *Activities I've Given Up On*, take some time to think about and write down those activities that used to give you a sense of accomplishment or enjoyment but are no longer part of your daily life. The goal is to gradually return to making those former activities part of your everyday routine.

At this point, you may be thinking, "I'm depressed. I don't feel like doing those things, and I won't enjoy them anyway." You are partially right. You probably will not feel like doing the things your therapist thinks will be helpful for you to do. For example, perhaps you once enjoyed the hobby of painting, and your therapist thinks it would be helpful to do some painting a few times a week. If you are like most people with depression, you might make the common mistake of thinking that you first have to *feel* like painting before you can *do* it.

With depression, the reality is that it is the other way around. The first step is *doing*. Start painting, even if you do not feel like it. You may think it is going to be awful, and that is okay for now. If you are willing to try painting and pay close attention to how you are feeling while you are doing it, you will notice that it is not as awful as you expected. After you finish painting, you may notice that you feel somewhat better than if you had not tried at all.

If you stick with it, you will eventually start to feel like painting again because you anticipate that you will feel better afterward—but notice that the *doing* had to come before the *feeling*. It is okay to start slowly. Set modest goals for yourself, and see how it goes. For example, you can start with 10 minutes of painting and gradually increase from there. With the help of your therapist, use Worksheet 6: *Making Good Things Happen Again* to set a modest goal for yourself.

After you complete your planned activity, you may determine that you *do not* feel better, and that is okay too. Even if you do not feel better, stick with it, and remind yourself that you accomplished something that was difficult. The next time you try it, the outcome may be better—but you will never know unless you try.

This chapter helps get you started on some activities that can provide important opportunities to experience positive emotions—things such as pride, satisfaction, and pleasure—in your daily life. Although we will be moving on to other important topics in the chapters that follow, your work on these activities can continue. Review Worksheet 5 every week or two, and set goals for reintroducing those activities into your daily life. Use Worksheet 6 to select specific activities. After you have started doing them, keep them up! For example, if you set a goal one week to play basketball at the gym for an hour, do it again the next week, and the next, and so on. The idea is not just to cross an activity off your list but to make the activities a routine part of your life.

A common reaction to the idea of reintroducing pleasant activities that are for your own benefit and enjoyment is concern about time constraints. You may find yourself thinking, "I do not have time for these things. I don't even have time for the things that I *have* to do!" If so, you are probably someone who would benefit from focusing on your *wants* rather than only on your *shoulds*. These activities do not have to take up a lot of your time to be helpful. If you do not have an hour to walk in the park, how about 10 minutes to walk around your neighborhood? Your therapist can help you set reasonable activity goals if you find that you are struggling.

Worksheet 4: My Daily Activities

Time	Day 1	Day 2	Day 3
8:00 AM			
9:00 AM			
10:00 AM			
11:00 AM			
12:00 PM			
1:00 PM			
2:00 PM			
3:00 PM			
4:00 PM			
5:00 PM			
6:00 PM			
7:00 PM			
8:00 PM			
9:00 PM			
10:00 PM			
11:00 PM			
12:00 AM			

Time	Day 4	Day 5	Day 6
8:00 AM			
9:00 AM			
10:00 AM			
11:00 AM			
12:00 PM			
1:00 PM			
2:00 PM			
3:00 PM			
4:00 PM			
5:00 PM			
6:00 PM			
7:00 PM			
8:00 PM			
9:00 PM			
10:00 PM			
11:00 PM			
12:00 AM			

Worksheet 5: Activities I've Given Up On

Use this worksheet to generate a list of *goal-directed, pleasurable, or rewarding activities* that you have given up on or decreased since you became depressed. Think about activities that you do not do anymore (or not as often as before) but used to enjoy or find satisfying. You may include activities that you have often thought about doing and would like to do but have never actually tried. List as many as you can think of at this time.

Activities you have given up on or do not do as often as you used to:

1. _____

2. _____

3. _____

4. _____

5. _____

6. _____

7. _____

8. _____

9. _____

10. _____

Worksheet 6: Making Good Things Happen Again

With help from your therapist, select an activity to start or increase over the next week. Write down specific goals and plans for this activity. Make copies of this sheet, and use a separate one for each activity you plan to work on. You will continue to use this sheet each week as you plan additional activities. Remember to set reasonable expectations and goals!

Planned activity: _____

What good things may happen if you do this?	
How many times will you do the activity and for how long and when (be specific)?	
What is likely to get in the way (obstacles)?	
How will you deal with these obstacles?	
(After doing the activity) *How did it go? How did you feel?*	

Earlier when you talked with your therapist about important people in your life, that conversation (and the information gathered in Worksheet 3) included questions about what those people expect from you. You spent some time thinking about the *standards* those people have for you and what happens when you do not live up to their standards and expectations. You also have expectations and standards for yourself. Together, your own standards and the standards that come from other people are characteristics that define the person you are striving to be. Desired characteristics can fall into two categories:

1. *Ideal self-guides* are characteristics that you would ideally like to have.
2. *Ought self-guides* are characteristics that you think you ought to (or should) have.

Your Ideal and Ought Self-Guides

How can you tell the difference between your ideal and ought self-guides? When you consider ought self-guides, think of your *shoulds*, those characteristics that are concerned with your responsibilities and obligations. The following are some examples of ought self-guides:

- Being reliable (e.g., following through with promises, showing up for required meetings or appointments)
- Being honest (e.g., not lying to a spouse or partner, admitting mistakes)
- Being a provider for your family (e.g., holding down a steady job, paying for your children's education)

While reading about these shoulds, you might have sensed a connection between ought self-guides and prevention goals. We use prevention goals as a way of keeping up with responsibilities and obligations. If we are living up to our ought standards, we are keeping unpleasant things from happening. Using the previous examples, being reliable could mean preventing people from getting angry with you; being honest could mean preventing being embarrassed by getting caught in a lie; and being a provider could mean preventing foreclosure on a home.

> Ought self-guides are concerned with responsibilities and obligations (i.e., shoulds) and are connected to prevention goals.

When you think of your ideal self-guides, think of your *wants* or *desires*, characteristics that are concerned with your aspirations or accomplishments. The following are examples of ideal self-guides:

- Being a master gardener
- Being witty (i.e., being able to think on the spot and make humorous comments)
- Being knowledgeable about current events (e.g., reading the paper, watching the news)

Notice that in contrast to the ought self-guides, if you fail when it comes to these ideal characteristics, there are typically no dire outcomes. Failing at being witty is not going to have serious concrete consequences such as losing a job or house. However, it can lead to disappointment, which you may remember is a consequence of failing at promotion goals. These ideal self-guides are connected to promotion goals. We use promotion goals as a way of trying to become the person we ideally want to be.

> Ideal self-guides are concerned with aspirations and accomplishments (i.e., desires) and are connected with promotion goals.

Your Self-System and Self-Discrepancies

You have many different standards—ideal and ought self-guides, standards you have for yourself, and expectations that other people have for you. You are doing quite well with some of these expectations and standards, but you may be struggling with others. Maybe you are consistently honest and reliable, for example, but you wish you could be better at keeping up with current events. How do you know whether you are doing well? You make comparisons between who you are (which we refer to as your *self-beliefs*) and your self-guides.

> **Self-beliefs are characteristics that describe the person you actually are.**

These comparisons usually are not done intentionally. Most people do not sit down at the kitchen table every week and spend time thinking about who they are and who they want to be. You may not be aware of making the comparisons, but you probably are aware of their consequences. For example, when you think to yourself, "I need to work on getting to my appointments on time," that is the end product of a comparison between your actual self (i.e., someone who is chronically late) and your ought self-guide (i.e., being someone who is usually on time to appointments).

> **Self-discrepancy is a mismatch between the person you are (i.e., self-belief) and the person you want to be (i.e., ideal self-guide) or the person you think you should be (i.e., ought self-guide).**

When you find that you need to work on some goal because you think you could do better, you have spotted a *self-discrepancy*. A self-discrepancy means that you are not meeting a certain expectation you have for yourself or not meeting expectations that other people have for you. These discrepancies can be useful signals. They can motivate us to make changes or focus on doing something better, such as setting a goal of planning ahead to get to appointments on time; this is effective self-regulation.

People who are depressed often have self-discrepancies but have trouble making changes or doing things differently to reduce those discrepancies. When self-regulation is not working properly, self-discrepancies remain, and nothing changes, making the depression worse.

As you have been reading about your self-beliefs and ideal and ought self-guides, you may have been thinking about the characteristics that you would include in those categories to describe yourself. It helps to write those things down so that you and your therapist can better understand the ways in which you are struggling to be the kind of person you want to be. Worksheet 7: *Learning About My Self-Guides and Self-Beliefs* walks you through the process of identifying your self-beliefs and self-guides and uncovering your self-discrepancies. The worksheet should be completed primarily in session with the help of your therapist. However, your therapist may ask you to do some additional work on it at home.

Some people find it difficult to complete Worksheet 7, and if that is your experience, you are not alone. Many people do not often spend time thinking about how to describe themselves, and this process can be challenging. After you start thinking about these aspects of yourself, especially your ideal and ought selves, you may find that you continue to think about them. For example, you may start to notice that *who you are, who you should be*, and *who you want to be* change depending on the situation (e.g., at home, out with friends, biking on a trail). You may come up with new characteristics that you had not thought about before. If so, share them with your therapist, and add them to Worksheet 7. You will be using this information as you move on in the program.

Worksheet 7: Learning About My Self-Guides and Self-Beliefs

NOTE: THIS WORKSHEET SHOULD BE COMPLETED IN SESSION WITH THE HELP OF YOUR THERAPIST.

> *Remember*:
>
> Your **actual self-beliefs** are your beliefs concerning the attributes or characteristics you think you *actually* possess. In other words, what kind of person do you think you actually are?

List the attributes or characteristics that describe the kind of person you think you actually are. Start by listing your characteristics, and then review them and indicate how well each characteristic describes you on a scale of 1 (does not describe me well at all) to 10 (describes me extremely well).

Characteristics of your actual self	How well it describes you
1. _____	_____
2. _____	_____
3. _____	_____
4. _____	_____
5. _____	_____
6. _____	_____
7. _____	_____
8. _____	_____
9. _____	_____
10. _____	_____

> *Remember*:
>
> Your **ideal self-guides** are your beliefs concerning the attributes or characteristics *you ideally would like to* possess. In other words, what kind of person do you ideally want to be to reach your aspirations?

List the attributes or characteristics that describe the kind of person you would *ideally* like to be. Start by listing your characteristics, and then review them and indicate how important each characteristic is to you on a scale of 1 (not at all important) to 10 (extremely important).

Characteristics of your ideal self	Importance
1. _____	_____
2. _____	_____
3. _____	_____
4. _____	_____
5. _____	_____
6. _____	_____
7. _____	_____
8. _____	_____
9. _____	_____
10. _____	_____

Remember:

Your **ought self-guides** are your beliefs concerning the attributes or characteristics *you believe you should* possess. In other words, what kind of person do you believe you should be in order to fulfill your duties or obligations?

List the attributes or characteristics that describe the kind of person you believe you *ought* to be. Start by listing your characteristics, and then review them and indicate how important each characteristic is to you on a scale of 1 (not at all important) to 10 (extremely important).

Characteristics of your ought self   **Importance**

1. _____   _____

2. _____   _____

3. _____   _____

4. _____   _____

5. _____   _____

6. _____   _____

7. _____   _____

8. _____   _____

9. _____   _____

10. _____   _____

By now, you have become familiar with many of the pieces that make up your self-regulatory style. You have explored your self-beliefs (i.e., actual self), your self-guides (your standards for yourself as well as the expectations that other people have of you), and your promotion and prevention goals. You also learned about self-discrepancies and how they can motivate you or, especially in the case of depression, make you feel defeated and self-critical.

Self-regulation does not happen only during a therapy session or at home when thinking about a therapy assignment—it happens in real life! When you got up yesterday morning, you had some goals in mind, although you probably did not think about them as goals. You might have thought, "I really need to remember to pay that utility bill today so I don't end up with a late fee." That is a prevention goal. Maybe you had plans to get together with a friend for lunch—which sounds like a promotion goal (i.e., making something good happen), right? Well, it depends. Maybe you did not feel like being social, but you went anyway because you knew that otherwise your friend be angry. If that was the main reason you did not cancel the lunch date, you were focused on preventing an unpleasant outcome (i.e., a prevention goal).

Monitoring Daily Situations: What Was My Goal?

Goal 2 of this phase of self-system therapy focuses on exploring how you pursue your goals as you go about your regular daily activities. You will be asking yourself over and over, "What was my goal in that situation? What was I trying to accomplish?" Many possible goals can come up in any situation. Sometimes you have to think very carefully about the *why* question to figure out which goal was in the driver's seat. *Why* did you decide not to cancel your lunch even though you wanted to? If it was because you did not want your friend to be mad, your goal was focused on prevention. If it was because you typically enjoy spending time with that person, your goal was focused on promotion. Sometimes it is difficult to figure out what your goal was, and your therapist is there to help you out.

Looking at how you approach different situations in your daily life is a very important part of this treatment program. You and your therapist will use this information to identify common themes in your everyday experiences—consistencies in the ways that you set and pursue goals, in how much your efforts pay off, and, importantly, in what does not seem to be working well for you in various situations. Make lots of copies of Worksheet 8 (*Examining Current Situations*) and Worksheet 10 (*Examining My Standards and Self-Beliefs*) because you will be keeping track of a number of situations over the next several weeks. You will also use Worksheets 9 and 11, respectively, to discover common themes in your situations and in your standards and self-beliefs.

There are four steps in this exploration process, which also is called psychological situation analysis (PSA). The first two steps are

1. **Examine current situations (Worksheet 8):** Focusing on the most important or most emotional experiences of each day, think about what your goal was (promotion or prevention), what you did (how you acted or handled the situation), and the outcome (how other people responded and how you felt afterward). An example of Worksheet 8 is provided to show what the answers to these questions might look like for a hypothetical situation.
2. **Identify common themes from those situations (Worksheet 9):** After you have analyzed many situations from step 1, what do you notice across those situations about your goals, your actions, and the outcomes?

Monitoring Daily Situations: What Were My Standards or Self-Beliefs?

The second part of the PSA involves asking you to think about what standards (i.e., ideal and ought self-guides) and self-beliefs (i.e., characteristics of your actual self) apply to your everyday situations. In Chapter 5, you began a list of those self-guides and self-beliefs. Use that list for this part of the PSA. You may also discover other standards and beliefs, ones you had not thought of before. It is helpful for you and your therapist to add new ones along the way.

How do you determine which standards or self-beliefs apply? To demonstrate, say you are enrolled in a class at your local community college and are required to complete a group project that makes up 40% of the final grade. Two days before the project is due, one of the group members calls you, says that because some things have come up at work he cannot complete his part, and asks you to do it for him. One of your self-beliefs is that you are a responsible and conscientious person, so that belief definitely applies here. However, one of your standards for yourself is that you do not let others take advantage of you, and that one also applies. As this example shows, more than one self-belief or standard can apply to a situation, and it is important to include all of them on your worksheets.

Here are the last two steps of the PSA:

3. **Examine your standards in current situations (Worksheet 10):** In this step, you will continue what you did in step 1, but you will also consider the standards and self-guides that apply in your current situations. Again, an example is included to show what a completed sheet might look like for a hypothetical situation.

4. **Identify common themes in your standards (Worksheet 11):** After you have analyzed situations from step 3, what do you notice across those situations about your standards? Again, an example is included.

Throughout this program, you will hear a common refrain from your therapist: What was your goal? This simple question is a very powerful one for many people. Our motives for acting the way we do, or for making the decisions that we make, are strongly connected to how we feel emotionally and how we view ourselves.

The aim of this chapter is to help you start making a habit of asking one question: What was my goal? Even when you do not have a worksheet in front of you, try to remember to ask yourself this question as you go about your daily life. Continue to notice patterns or common themes, as you did in Worksheets 9 and 11, and if you notice something new, share it with your therapist.

Worksheet 8: Examining Current Situations (Example)

This worksheet is designed to help you practice taking a closer look at situations from your day-to-day life. Here is an example so you can see how to fill it out.

Briefly describe the situation.	I asked a coworker to take one of my work shifts in 2 weeks.
Your *goals* in the situation: What were you trying to *accomplish* or *avoid*?	Goal: to find someone to fill in for me at work so that I could go to an appointment; I was trying to <u>avoid</u> having to reschedule the appointment because I would have to wait months to get in.
What did you *do* in the situation to pursue your goals?	I sent the coworker a text.
What was the outcome? How did the other people respond?	She didn't respond at all.
How did you feel afterward?	Anxious and confused.

Worksheet 8: Examining Current Situations

Now it is your turn. Focus on the *most important or most emotional* experiences that happened during your day. For each experience, fill in all of the boxes. Make copies of this worksheet, and keep a record of each experience on a different sheet.

Briefly describe the situation.	
Your *goals* in the situation: What were you trying to *accomplish* or *avoid*?	
What did you *do* in the situation to pursue your goals?	
What was the outcome? How did the other people respond?	
How did you feel afterward?	

Worksheet 9: Common Themes in My Situations

Review the situations you have described using Worksheet 8, and answer the following questions as best you can. You and your therapist will compare notes.

What common themes did you find regarding **your goals***?*

_____

_____

_____

_____

What common themes did you find regarding **how you tried to pursue these goals***?*

_____

_____

_____

_____

What common themes did you find regarding the outcomes or **how people responded to you***?*

_____

_____

_____

_____

What common themes did you find regarding **how you felt afterward***?*

_____

_____

_____

_____

Worksheet 10: Examining My Standards and Self-Beliefs (Example)

This worksheet is similar to Worksheet 8, but with additional questions about which of your standards or self-beliefs apply. Here is an example of a worksheet that has already been completed.

Briefly describe the situation.	My girlfriend and I had a fight about moving into a different apartment complex.
Your *goals* in the situation: What were you trying to *accomplish* or *avoid*?	I really want to move so that we can be closer to a nice park and walking trail, which I would enjoy (<u>accomplish</u>).
What did you *do* in the situation to pursue your goals?	I said I would not renew our current lease.
What was the outcome? How did the other people respond?	She got mad when I refused to renew the lease and became even more adamant about not moving to the place I want.
How did you feel afterward?	Disappointed, irritated
What standards or self-beliefs apply to this situation?	Standard: I should be in control of every situation.
Did the standards or self-beliefs come from you or someone else (and who)?	"Being controlling" is what my father expected of me.

Worksheet 10: Examining My Standards and Self-Beliefs

Now it is your turn. Focus on the *most important* or *most emotional* experiences that happen during your day. For each experience, fill in all of the boxes. Make copies of this worksheet, and keep a record of each experience on a different sheet.

Briefly describe the situation.	
Your *goals* in the situation: What were you trying to *accomplish* or *avoid*?	
What did you *do* in the situation to pursue your goals?	
What was the outcome? How did the other people respond?	
How did you feel afterward?	
What standards or self-beliefs apply to this situation?	
Did the standards or self-beliefs come from you or someone else (and who)?	

Worksheet 11: Common Themes: My Standards and Self-Beliefs (Example)

Review the situations and standards from Worksheet 10. As you practiced identifying your standards (or the standards that other people hold for you) and your self-beliefs in particular situations, you may have noticed some common themes across your experiences. This worksheet can help you summarize what you have learned. Here is a worksheet with a few example entries.

Self-guide or self-belief	When did you adopt it?	Is it yours or someone else's?	Does it help you or get in the way? How?	When does it come up (what situations)?
Being the top student in all my classes (self-guide)	Grade school (probably 3rd grade)	My parents always expected this of me. When I think about it, it isn't all that important to me.	It does help me try my hardest, but if my hardest doesn't result in the top grade, I feel worthless. I get so focused on the grade that I lose sight of what I am learning.	Any situation related to school or work
Being the peacekeeper in my family (self-belief)	Probably when I was a teenager	Mine	It's a lot of pressure to put on myself. I can't control other people's behavior, and it just frustrates me. I don't see how it benefits me.	Any time there is conflict among members of my family
Being in a perfect relationship (self-guide)	When I started to see my friends getting married	Mine	It's not helpful at all. I compare my relationships (or lack thereof) to everyone else's and feel disappointed.	Any time I see a happy couple—out in public, on television, people I know

Worksheet 11: Common Themes: My Standards and Self-Beliefs

Now it is your turn. Your blank worksheet is longer than the example, and you may need even more space than what is provided. If so, make additional copies. Some people need more space, and others need less—there are no strict rules.

Self-guide or self-belief	When did you adopt it?	Is it yours or someone else's?	Does it help you or get in the way? How?	When does it come up (what situations)?

By now, you and your therapist have identified some clear areas related to your self-regulatory style that would be helpful to work on and that will be the focus from here on. In Chapters 7, 8, and 9 of this workbook, there are a number of strategies that your therapist may use, depending on what would be most helpful for you. Because your therapist will tailor these strategies to meet your needs, not everything in each chapter will apply to you.

Your therapist will choose the most effective strategies for you and may cover the material in these chapters out of order. You may address some or all of the goals in those chapters, and you may do them out of order. The program is designed to allow for that kind of flexibility.

Most people with depression can benefit from working on reducing self-discrepancies. We mentioned in Chapter 5 that depression typically involves self-discrepancies that seem to stick around without any progress being made. You may have noticed some of these when you were analyzing your daily situations. Were there self-guides (i.e., ideals or oughts) that kept coming up in situations in which you felt upset or disappointed in yourself? If so, those are the kind of chronic self-discrepancies that need to be addressed.

Reducing Self-Discrepancies: Clearing Your Hurdles

Self-discrepancies can be reduced (or eliminated) in several ways. When it comes to reducing self-discrepancies, imagine yourself as a hurdler, and the discrepancies are like hurdles that you are unable to clear. What could you do to solve that problem? A simple solution is to lower the height of the hurdle, which is like lowering your standard (ought or ideal self-guide). Maybe the reason you cannot clear the bar (i.e., achieve your standard) is that it is too high, and, no matter how hard you try, you will never clear it. With the bar set lower, you can clear the hurdles. Because your standards are lowered, the discrepancy is no longer a problem. In Worksheet 12: *Revising My Standards or Expectations*, you will carefully evaluate some of those standards.

Reducing Self-Discrepancies: Taking a New Approach

Returning to our hurdler analogy, another strategy for trying to clear your high hurdles is to change your training routine, perhaps by adding new hurdle drills or sprint training. Similarly, when it comes to self-discrepancies, you may look for new ways to approach your goal, perhaps by learning a new skill or changing the environment in which your goal is pursued. With this option, you do not lower your standards. With time and commitment, the new approach will allow you to meet your expectations.

If you cannot seem to clear the hurdles no matter what you do, you may decide that hurdling just is not for you and start focusing your physical and mental energy on something else such as biking in the park. Some self-discrepancies may have taken on an exaggerated sense of importance in your life. You may not want or be able to abandon those standards completely (some hurdles should not be avoided), but you may be better off if they did not have such a central focus in your life. For example, maybe you have struggled your whole life with low self-confidence and you constantly berate yourself for not exuding the kind of self-confidence you think others have. One approach is to recognize this barrier and then decide that your inner lack of confidence is really not the most important thing in your life and does not define who you are as a person. Instead of focusing on trying to increase your confidence, you focus on your strengths and on making sure your lack of confidence does not get in the way of the things you want to do.

Sometimes, when self-discrepancies become exaggerated, they cloud our vision of ourselves. We can become so focused on the ways we do not measure up that we lose sight of all the ways in which we do. Worksheets 13 (*Getting in Touch with My Positive Qualities*), 14 (*How Do My Positive*

Qualities Hide?), and 15 (*Unhiding My Positive Qualities*) can help you see yourself more clearly by getting you to pay more attention to your strengths and positive qualities.

This chapter focuses on helping you bring your self-guides and self-beliefs more in line with each other. Keep in mind that this kind of change will not happen overnight. In Chapter 3, you explored some of your most important relationships and how they shaped the standards and expectations you have for yourself. Some of the relationships you explored probably originated in your childhood, and the standards and expectations related to them are longstanding. Until now, you probably never questioned them. The same is true for your self-beliefs; you have spent a lifetime developing your view of yourself, and maybe no one has ever challenged that view. As with any new skill, learning to adjust your standards and to adopt a more balanced view of yourself will take effort and practice. Stick with it, and your efforts will pay off!

Worksheet 12: Revising My Standards or Expectations

Some of your standards or expectations may be getting in your way rather than helping to motivate you. This worksheet helps you to examine your standards and revise them. Use one worksheet per standard, and make additional copies as needed.

Your current standard or expectation:

_____

Does this standard involve making good things happen or preventing bad things from happening? In other words, is it related to how you want to be or how you feel you should be?

_____

_____

_____

Where do you think this standard came from? Is it important to you or to other people, or both?

_____

_____

_____

What does it mean to meet this standard? What are the specific expectations, and what must you do to meet them? How do you know whether you are meeting them?

_____

_____

_____

Is it possible to meet and maintain this standard? If so, how much effort does it take?

_____

_____

_____

What happens when you are able to live up to this standard or expectation?

_____

_____

_____

What happens when you are unable to live up to this standard or expectation?

_____

_____

_____

How could you change or replace this standard (or expectation) to make it a hurdle you could clear more easily?

_____

_____

_____

Your revised standard or expectation:

_____

If you adopted this revised (or new) standard or expectation, how would your life be better?

_____

_____

_____

If you adopted this revised (or new) standard or expectation, how would your life be worse?

_____

_____

_____

Are you willing to try adopting this new standard as an experiment for a short period? Decide how long you are willing to try it (e.g., 2 weeks), and record the results of your experiment below. When thinking about the outcomes, consider the practical consequences, the effects it had on other people, and how you felt.

What went well (positive outcomes)?	What didn't go well (negative outcomes)?
How did these results compare with what you expected?	

Worksheet 13: Getting in Touch with My Positive Qualities

In the space below, list your positive qualities or strengths (e.g., compassion, sense of humor, loyalty, reliability), and give an example of a recent situation in which that quality applied.

Your positive quality	Sample situation

Worksheet 14: How Do My Positive Qualities Hide?

You may have had a hard time completing Worksheet 13. Your strengths and positive qualities are definitely there, but depression has a way of keeping them hidden from your view. The following questions can help you think about out how your positive qualities hide.

How difficult was it for you to make the list of positive qualities in Worksheet 13? Did you find yourself minimizing your positive qualities or thinking that they were not important?

_____

_____

_____

_____

Have friends or family members complimented you for having a quality that you do not see in yourself? For example, you may hear a friend describe you as generous and be surprised to hear it. Provide your own examples here.

_____

_____

_____

_____

What kinds of thoughts interfere with being able to appreciate your positive qualities? For example, you may discount generous behaviors by telling yourself that "anyone would do the same thing."

_____

_____

_____

_____

What ways of thinking could help you more easily recognize your positive qualities and give them the weight they deserve? For example, you may remind yourself that not everyone is generous and that your willingness to do things for others means a lot to them.

_____

_____

_____

_____

Think about times when you notice the positive qualities you listed in Worksheet 13. Which situations are most likely to trigger positive thoughts about yourself? Are there certain people in your life around whom you generally feel pleased with yourself?

_____

_____

_____

_____

Think about situations in which you rarely see yourself in a positive way. Which situations are least likely to trigger positive thoughts about yourself? Are there certain people in your life around whom you generally do not feel pleased with yourself?

_____

_____

_____

_____

Worksheet 15: Unhiding My Positive Qualities

Another way to unhide (i.e., uncover) your positive qualities is to do things that allow your strengths to be seen. With help from your therapist, you can plan activities that bring out your positive qualities so that you can see them more clearly.

Your assignment: What can you do to uncover your strengths?

_____

_____

_____

_____

What is likely to get in the way (i.e., obstacles)?

_____

_____

_____

_____

How will you deal with these obstacles?

_____

_____

_____

_____

(After completing the assignment:) What positive qualities in yourself came up during the assignment?

_____

_____

_____

_____

(After completing the assignment:) Overall, how did it go? How did the actual outcome compare with what you expected?

_____

_____

_____

_____

This chapter focuses on improving how you go about pursuing your goals. Two strategies are used. These strategies will help you think about and act on your goals more effectively and will give you more opportunities to experience positive emotions in your daily life. The first strategy looks at how you set and pursue your goals. For goals that are a struggle for you, adjustments can be made in how you define the goals and in the strategies you use to pursue them; this can help you improve your progress. The second strategy involves looking at your tendency to focus on promotion or prevention goals. If the balance between promotion and prevention goals is off, you can tip the scale back in the right direction.

Defining Your Goals

Redefining goals and adjusting the strategies you use to pursue goals can help you be more effective. The first part of this chapter focuses on the steps needed to set clear and realistic goals and to plan effective strategies for making progress toward those goals.

The first step in effective goal pursuit is to make sure your expectations are reasonable and achievable; in other words, it is important that you set *realistic* goals. In Chapter 2, we talked about the fact that goals that are very abstract are difficult to work with. For example, one of your goals may be to be a good parent. The problem with this goal is that the definition can change from day to day. Today, being a good parent might mean taking your child to a pediatrician appointment and comforting him during the visit. Tomorrow it might mean arranging a play date.

This type of abstract goal is a common one, but it implies that if you are not being a good parent, you must be a bad one. There is no middle ground. Moreover, because this type of goal is vague, it is hard to tell whether you are making progress. What measuring stick can be used to determine how good you are as a parent? Without a ruler of some sort, it is difficult to tell where you stand or how far you need to go.

Wanting to be a good parent—whatever than means to you—is reasonable, but it would be easier to know how you are doing in that area if your goal were more specific and concrete. For example, you can define being a good parent in part as teaching your children about their familial and cultural background. This is more specific, but we can do better. A clearer and more observable goal might be to make sure that your children spend time with their grandparents at least four times per year so that they can learn about their grandparents' history and experiences. This goal is better because it is much more well-defined. If you arrange for four visits per year, you have achieved your goal. If you can only get in three visits, you are 75% of the way there!

Making a goal more specific sometimes requires breaking it down into smaller parts. For example, a goal of having a nice yard probably involves a number of steps. Instead of focusing on the nice yard, which may feel rather overwhelming, you could focus on a series of smaller goals. First, focus on cleaning up debris and pulling weeds. Second, work on trimming back branches and bushes. Third, replace mulch in the planting beds. Each of these steps could be broken down even further. Maybe you have only 30 minutes on the weekend to devote to the yard, so you can start with cleaning up the debris in one section of the front yard only.

In addition to making goals more specific and concrete, you can make a goal more realistic by changing certain elements of it. For example, you can change the time frame. Maybe you have decided that you want to save enough money to take a trip this summer, but unexpected expenses keep popping up, and it is taking longer to save than you had expected. Delaying the trip until the following summer may be more realistic and may reduce your disappointment and frustration.

In some cases, there may be some other goal that you need to focus on first. For example, perhaps you had a falling out with a friend, but you really miss that person and want to get back to the way things were. Your primary goal of repairing that relationship may involve many steps, and it may be helpful to focus first on a more modest goal, such as simply reestablishing contact.

Worksheet 16: *Setting Realistic Goals* can help you determine whether your goals are realistic and well-defined. When you are struggling with a goal, it is often helpful to go back to the drawing board and evaluate the extent to which the goal is a reasonable one to begin with. If you start with an unrealistic goal, you may be setting yourself up for failure right out of the gate. Having an outsider's perspective on your goals is often helpful, and your therapist can help you evaluate the extent to which your goals are realistic.

Strategies for Making Progress

After you have a goal that is concrete and realistic, coming up with a well-considered plan for how to start working on the goal is the next step. Worksheet 17: *Evaluating How I Pursue My Goals* asks you to think about a goal you have had some difficulty with. Evaluate the strategies you have tried in the past—what worked and what did not work? Think about different ways of approaching that goal—what other strategies or routes could you take that might be more effective?

Sometimes when it comes to thinking about goal pursuit strategies, we can get tunnel vision. We can only see one way to approach a goal and have a hard time seeing other possibilities. If you are having this problem, it is often helpful to get input from other people. Your therapist may have some ideas, but also think about supportive family members, friends, fellow students, or colleagues at work. Be careful not to immediately dismiss ideas that seem silly or unrealistic; sometimes being open to different approaches can really pay off! Talking with other people and brainstorming ideas can help to reduce your tunnel vision.

Shifting the Balance: Promotion and Prevention Focus

Earlier in this program, you monitored your goals and standards during everyday situations. You and your therapist then discussed common themes that emerged from those situations. The first question on Worksheet 9 asked what you learned about your goals in everyday situations. If you are like many people struggling with depression, you probably observed that you did not have many promotion goals—in other words, you did not often try to engage in pleasurable activities and experiences, things that are intended for your own enjoyment or sense of accomplishment.

You and your therapist have been working on correcting the imbalance between promotion and prevention. In Chapter 4, you started by looking at your daily activities, taking special notice of what was missing from your regular routine. You also started trying to increase pleasant activities (i.e., promotion-focused behavior) each week, which is a great way of shifting the balance so that you have more opportunities to experience the sense of accomplishment and pleasure that goes along with making progress on promotion goals.

Using Worksheet 18 (*Promotion and Prevention—What's My Focus?*), you will now be asked to reflect on what you have learned about your overall tendency to focus on promotion or prevention. Do you have a balance of promotion and prevention activities in your life, or are the scales usually tipped too far in favor of one or the other? On Worksheet 19 (*Promotion and Prevention—Changing My Focus*), you are asked to consider the costs and benefits of promotion and prevention and to step outside of your comfort zone by trying to adopt a different focus in some situations. For example, if you tend to have a prevention focus when talking to a certain family member (e.g., making sure you do not make that person angry), you might consider focusing on a different goal (e.g., trying to learn something new about that person in order to strengthen your relationship).

In Chapter 7, we pointed out that changing your self-guides and self-beliefs does not happen overnight, and the same is true of the changes you have worked on in this chapter. If you are like many people who struggle with depression and anxiety, your scale may be tipped toward prevention goals in many situations. The goal in this program is not to flip the scales in the opposite direction—that would be an extremely unrealistic goal! Instead, the goal is to make you aware of your tendency and to get you to think about the possibility that focusing solely on prevention goals may not be the best fit for every situation. Recall from Chapter 2 that promotion and prevention goals are both important—it is all about balance!

You may have goals that you have had difficulty reaching, or perhaps you are trying to set a new goal for yourself. This worksheet can help you decide whether a particular goal is realistic; if not, it can help you think about how to revise your goal. Make extra copies of this worksheet, and use one for each goal you want to evaluate.

Initial Goal: _____

STEP 1: How *realistic* is this goal?

Is reaching this goal possible? If a friend told you that this was his or her goal, how realistic do you think it would be for that person?

_____

_____

_____

_____

Do you have the resources or skills needed to reach the goal?

_____

_____

_____

_____

Are there obstacles beyond your control that would prevent you from reaching this goal? (For example, if your goal is to get a raise, but your boss is incredibly stingy, it will be difficult to reach your goal no matter how well you perform at your job.)

_____

_____

_____

_____

STEP 2: If your goal is **not** realistic, try revising it by thinking through the following questions.

If the goal is too overwhelming, can it be broken into smaller parts?

_____

_____

_____

_____

Is there a more immediate goal that could be reached first? (For example, do you need to get the car fixed before starting holiday shopping?)

_____

_____

_____

_____

Would the goal be more realistic if you developed additional skills before pursuing it?

_____

_____

_____

_____

Would the goal be more realistic if you changed a specific part of it?

_____

_____

_____

_____

Revised goal: _____

Repeat step 1 to be sure the goal is realistic; if not, try revising it again.

After you start working on this goal, how will you know you are making progress?

_____

_____

_____

_____

Worksheet 17: Evaluating How I Pursue My Goals

In Worksheet 16, you evaluated a goal that you have been having difficulty reaching or a new goal that you would like to start working on. The next step is to look at how to start making progress. This worksheet is designed to help you evaluate your *strategies* for pursuing goals.

Write down one goal you have had difficulty reaching. Make sure you have completed Worksheet 16 first so that the goal you are working on is realistic.

Realistic Goal:

_____

What strategies have you tried to reach this goal?

_____

_____

_____

_____

What other strategies could you try? If you are having tunnel vision, brainstorm ideas with other people you trust. List your ideas:

_____

_____

_____

_____

Evaluate the ideas on your list. For each of the strategies you could try, what are the benefits and costs? Make copies of this sheet if you have more than four strategies.

Strategies	Benefits	Costs
Strategy 1		
Strategy 2		
Strategy 3		
Strategy 4		

Worksheet 18: Promotion and Prevention—What's My Focus?

Based on what you have learned so far, are you generally more focused on promotion (i.e., making good things happen) or prevention (i.e., keeping bad things from happening)?

_____

_____

_____

_____

Where do you think this tendency came from? How and when do you think this tendency started, and why did it work well for you at that time?

_____

_____

_____

_____

In what situations are you more likely to use a promotion focus (e.g., hobbies, interacting with loved ones, practicing a skill)?

_____

_____

_____

In what situations are you more likely to use a prevention focus (e.g., work, school, financial situations, interacting with certain people)?

_____

_____

_____

Worksheet 19: Promotion and Prevention—Changing My Focus

Thinking back on everything you have learned about yourself so far in this program, what are the costs and benefits to you of a *promotion focus*?

Benefits of a promotion focus	Costs of a promotion focus

Thinking back on everything you have learned about yourself so far in this program, what are the costs and benefits to you of a *prevention focus*?

Benefits of a prevention focus	Costs of a prevention focus

List some situations in which you tend to use a *prevention* focus but a *promotion* focus might be more beneficial or lead to a better outcome.

Situation 1 _____

_____

_____

_____

Situation 2 _____

_____

_____

_____

Situation 3 _____

_____

_____

_____

Situation 4 _____

_____

_____

_____

Circle one situation from the list in which you could try a promotion focus. How can you think about that situation differently so that you are focused on trying to make something pleasant happen?

_____

_____

_____

Do you anticipate any problems or difficulties with your plan to try a different focus in that situation? If so, describe them and what you can do to resolve them.

_____

_____

_____

After you have followed through with the plan and using the questions that follow, describe how your trial run turned out.

Did your new focus change the way you felt about the situation beforehand?

_____

_____

_____

Did it change how you felt afterward?

_____

_____

_____

Did it have an impact on what you did in the situation or on the outcome?

_____

_____

_____

_____

How did other people respond (if others were involved)?

_____

_____

_____

_____

Identifying Perfectionistic Standards

Many people with depression have standards that are extremely high—so high that it is almost impossible to reach them. You are probably familiar with the term *perfectionism*, which is quite common in depression. You may recognize some of these characteristics of perfectionism in yourself:

- Having extremely high standards for yourself
- Feeling that other people have extremely high expectations of you
- Being very self-critical (i.e., being very hard on yourself if you feel that you are not living up to your high standards)
- Feeling that other people will reject you or be very disappointed in you if you do not live up to their expectations

If some or all of these characteristics seem to fit you, your high standards may be getting in your way. Being perfectionistic does not necessarily mean having high standards or goals in all areas of life. For example, you may be highly perfectionistic when it comes to your home. You may insist on a spotless kitchen at all times and may not invite others into your home unless everything is in its place and the floors are freshly vacuumed. You may feel that others are judging you based on your ability to maintain a perfect home. However, at work, you may have no problem turning in a report that has a few typos or sending an email before re-reading it.

Worksheet 20: *Identifying Perfectionistic Standards* can help you and your therapist identify the areas in your life in which you do and do not have perfectionistic standards and goals. You will be asked to think about where those high standards came from, although you may not know, especially if you have held those standards for a very long time. Sometimes, people have a sense about the origins of their standards. For example, a perfectionistic housekeeper may have been raised in a household with similar high standards where compliance with those standards was instilled consistently throughout childhood. If you are not sure, leave that part of the worksheet blank, and discuss it with your therapist.

Modifying Perfectionistic Standards

People with perfectionistic standards often balk at the idea of lowering their standards. There is nothing wrong with striving for high standards and trying to be the best that you can be. However, when it comes to perfectionism, people are sometimes too rigid about their standards and too self-critical when they are unable to live up to them at all times. That is when trying to be the best that you can be is no longer working in your favor. Constantly beating yourself up over not being good enough is probably not how you want to live your life.

Have you noticed that you have a double standard when it comes to the perfectionistic areas in your life, such as the ones you identified in Worksheet 20? Maybe you feel it is okay for your brother or your neighbor to have weeds in the yard or peeling paint on the windows ("The neighbors are just busy" or "It doesn't matter—I love my brother, and he is a generous person"), whereas having overgrown bushes in *your* yard means that you are lazy, a poor housekeeper, and an embarrassment. Sound familiar?

You are willing to cut others some slack, but you may be reluctant to lower your own standards. However, if those goals and standards are not working for you, it is time to reevaluate them. Using Worksheet 21 (*Modifying Perfectionistic Standards*), your therapist will work with you to take a realistic view of your perfectionistic goals and standards and explore more moderate alternatives. For example, a more moderate version of the goal "I must keep my email inbox cleared at all times" is "I will clear out my email inbox twice each day." Worksheet 22 (*Modifying Perfectionistic Standards: Cost-Benefit Analysis*) asks you to consider the costs and benefits of keeping your existing perfectionistic standards and the costs and benefits of changing them. When you have identified an area of your life in which the costs of continuing to pursue a perfectionistic goal outweigh the benefits, or there are important potential benefits of adopting a different goal, Worksheet 23 (*Modifying Perfectionistic Standards: Trying Out New Standards*) will challenge you to try out a new, more realistic standard.

The worksheets in this chapter seem deceptively simple. However, if you are someone who struggles with perfectionism, you know that changing your standards is anything but simple. For that reason, it is important that you work closely with your therapist as you take a hard look at how your perfectionistic standards affect your daily life, your emotions, and your view of yourself. As with many of the changes discussed in this program, trying to get a handle on your high standards will take time.

You may not feel ready to change your standards in certain areas of your life—if so, that is okay. Your therapist can help you find an area in which change might be a little bit easier. As you start to see the benefits of those changes, you may find that you want to apply them to other areas of your life as well.

Worksheet 20: Identifying Perfectionistic Standards

Think about the areas in which you tend to be the *most* perfectionistic or have the highest standards and goals. For example, concerning family matters, do you feel you must always listen patiently to your children? To maintain your health, do you feel that you must go running 6 days per week? In the office, do you feel you must keep your email inbox cleared at all times? List five perfectionistic standards or goals that you have the most difficulty living up to.

1. _____

2. _____

3. _____

4. _____

5. _____

Where do you think these standards or goals came from? When did you learn them? Who gave you the idea they were important? How did you decide to adopt them?

_____

_____

_____

_____

Think about the areas in which you tend to be the *least* perfectionistic or have more moderate goals. For example, when providing meals, are you happy to use prepackaged meals or order takeout on a busy night? Concerning housekeeping, do you think that a few dust bunnies never hurt anyone? In maintaining your health, do you think, "I'll work out if I have time"? List five of your least perfectionistic standards or goals below:

1. _____

2. _____

3. _____

4. _____

5. _____

Where do you think these standards or goals came from? Why do you think it is easier for you to live with more moderate goals in these particular areas?

_____

_____

_____

_____

Worksheet 21: Modifying Perfectionistic Standards

Review the five most perfectionistic standards or goals you identified in Worksheet 20, and consider them as you answer the following questions. Make extra copies of this worksheet as needed, and use one worksheet for each standard or goal.

Perfectionistic Standard: _____

What are the specific behaviors or actions that define this standard?	
Name one person who consistently and fully lives up to this standard. How do you know?	
By your estimation, what percentage of people in the general population consistently and completely lives up to this standard?	
How likely is it that *you* can consistently and completely live up to this standard?	
Name someone who is successful even though he or she has *not* attained this standard.	

Worksheet 22: Modifying Perfectionistic Standards: Cost-Benefit Analysis

Create a revised, more moderate standard or goal for each perfectionistic one. This worksheet asks you to consider the costs and benefits of the perfectionistic and the more moderate standards.

Costs of perfectionistic standard or goal	*Benefits of perfectionistic standard or goal*

Costs of revised standard or goal	*Benefits of revised standard or goal*

Worksheet 23: Modifying Perfectionistic Standards: Trying Out New Standards

You have generated some moderate substitutes for your perfectionistic standards or goals. As an experiment, try one of them out for a week. During this "audition," pay attention to the practical consequences, your level of satisfaction with the substitute standard, and how you are thinking or feeling about yourself. Use this worksheet to keep track of your experiences.

New Standard Being Auditioned: _____

What were the practical consequences of aiming for the more moderate standard? For example, did it cause problems for your job or your family? Did others comment on the change? Did you have more time to spend on other things?

_____

_____

_____

_____

_____

How satisfied were you with this more moderate standard? Select one:

○ Not at all   ○ Somewhat   ○ A little   ○ Pretty   ○ Very   ○ Extremely
  satisfied   satisfied   satisfied   satisfied   satisfied   satisfied

How did you think or feel about yourself as a result of adopting the more moderate standard?

_____

_____

_____

_____

_____

CHAPTER 10

Concluding Treatment and Preventing Relapse

Congratulations on all of your hard work in this program so far! You and your therapist have learned a lot about self-regulation: your goals and standards, the strategies you use to pursue those goals, and how things typically turn out. You have also worked on making changes that can help you be more effective in certain difficult areas. One of your therapist's goals in this program has been to give you tools that allow you to continue to make progress on your own because your journey does not end here.

As you approach the end of this program, it is important to recognize the progress you have already made. Worksheet 24 (*Recognizing My Progress*) asks you to reflect on the changes you have made in how you handle a situation that is important to you. Do you think about the situation differently? Do you set different goals or have different standards? Do you handle it with new strategies? How has the outcome changed? Do you feel differently about the outcome? Do others react in new ways? Your therapist may also have noticed some changes that you did not notice or you forgot about, and you should add your therapist's observations to the worksheet as well.

It is important to make plans to keep your progress going. Self-regulation is a lifelong process for everyone, and you should expect to continue to ask yourself the questions that came up repeatedly throughout the course of therapy: *What is my goal? What kind of person do I want to be?* and *What kind of person do I think I should be?* Your answers to these questions will likely change over time, but for now, we want to focus on your most immediate goals. Worksheet 25 (*On My Own—Keeping My Progress Going*) can help you set realistic goals for your continued work after therapy and develop a plan for how to maintain your progress.

Maintaining Healthy Self-Regulation in Daily Life

We started this chapter by reviewing the progress you have made in this program and identifying the areas that you want to continue working on. However, even the most reasonable goal and carefully crafted plan are pointless if you never act on them. It can be difficult to stay motivated to work on your goals, and we recommend that you make it a point to focus on your goals as part of your regular daily routine. For example, you might take a few minutes to think about these things as you eat your breakfast or brush your teeth in the morning. Worksheets 26 and 27 can help you with this.

Worksheet 26 (*Being the Person I Want To Be*) asks you to identify one thing you want to work on each day. It might be a particular goal (e.g., "Help my cat get more exercise"), a behavior (e.g., "Spend less time on social media"), or a characteristic (e.g., "Be more assertive"). Make sure you choose something that is important to you and that can realistically be done that day, given other things you may have going on. Think about when and where you will have the opportunity to work on this goal, behavior, or characteristic. Because remembering to do it can be a big challenge, plan how you will remember (e.g., Will you set a reminder alarm on your phone? Will you leave yourself a Post-it note?)

Worksheet 27 (*Challenging Situations*) also involves thinking about something you want to work on during the day, but it focuses on challenging situations. Difficult situations will come up; there is no avoiding them. When you know you will be faced with a challenge, whether it is confronting a friend about a problem or navigating the first day at a new job, it helps to plan ahead and think about the things that are most important to you in those situations. You may not be able to avoid feeling stressed, but there are things you can do to feel satisfied with how you handle the situation. Worksheet 27 can be used on days when you know a challenging situation is coming.

It is normal and understandable to feel some anxiety and uncertainty about finishing therapy. Clients often have several concerns about what will happen and how they will handle things when they are on their own. Here we list and respond to several common questions and concerns that clients often raise at the end of therapy. You are encouraged to discuss your fears, worries, or doubts with your therapist. At the end of this chapter, we provide a worksheet that allows you to document specific plans recommended by your therapist that are tailored to your unique situation.

■ *I am afraid I will not be able to handle things on my own.*
  ■ One of the advantages of skills-based treatment programs such as this one is that the overall aim is to enable you to use the skills on your own. You and your therapist have been working on that goal all along, whether you realized it or not. You will probably be able to handle a lot more than you think you can, but there may be times when you struggle. You and your therapist will develop a plan (Worksheet 28: *Self-Monitoring and Coping After Therapy Ends*) so that you know exactly what to do if your own efforts do not seem to be working.

■ *What if I forget everything I learned?*
  ■ This workbook was designed specifically to help you remember what you have learned and continue to use it. You can refer to the workbook whenever you want to and have all the information at your fingertips. Make extra copies of the worksheets, and use them regularly.

■ *What if my depression comes back?*
  ■ That may happen. Depression is a recurrent condition, and many people experience more than one episode during their lifetime. The important thing is to monitor yourself so that when you feel things slipping, you can take action sooner rather than later. Using Worksheet 28, you and your therapist will create a monitoring plan that you can implement on your own. It will include a list of red flags—signs or symptoms that may indicate depression is coming back.

■ *What if something new goes wrong, something I have not worked on in therapy?*

■ The skills you learned in this program can be applied broadly to many different problems. You may find that it takes more effort to use your skills on a new problem, but it will probably feel satisfying if you are able to at least try. If you are feeling stuck and see one of those red flags, you have a plan in hand for what to do.

With a plan for how you will keep your progress going and how you will handle setbacks, you are ready to fly solo. You may not feel ready, and that is okay. Although you may feel anxious about ending therapy, it does not mean that something bad is going to happen. Do you recognize those worries as prevention focused? In this case, the prevention focus can be helpful if it gently reminds you that the end of therapy does not mean the work is done. As you proceed on your own, come back to this page frequently and ask yourself the following questions:

■ What are my standards or expectations for myself? What do others expect from me? Are those standards important to me, and are they reasonable?
■ Am I striving for a balance of promotion and prevention goals?
■ When I am unhappy or distressed about a particular situation, am I asking myself what my goal is?
■ Am I setting goals that are realistic, or am I setting myself up for failure?

If you find yourself falling short in any of these areas, remember that the chapters in this workbook can help you get back on track. The more you review the material and repeat the worksheets, the greater the likelihood that these skills will become second nature.

Worksheet 24: Recognizing My Progress

You and your therapist have discussed many situations in which you were struggling to reach important goals. As you get closer to completing therapy, it can be very helpful to see how your approach to reaching your goals *has changed* over time.

Briefly describe a common situation that is important to you (e.g., discussing a large purchase with your partner):

_____

_____

_____

_____

Your Old Approach

Describe how you handled this situation before you started therapy or early in therapy (e.g., you got angry and shut down when your partner did not agree with you).

Your old goals and expectations: _____

_____

_____

_____

What you said and did, and how you said and did it: _____

_____

_____

_____

The typical outcome (e.g., what happened, how you felt, how others reacted):

_____

_____

_____

_____

Your New Approach

Describe how you handled a similar situation recently (e.g., although you felt frustrated, you and your partner began to discuss compromises). Pay close attention to what is different now.

_____

Your NEW goals and expectations: _____

_____

_____

_____

What you RECENTLY said and did, and how you said and did it:

_____

_____

_____

_____

The outcome (e.g., what happened, how you felt, how others reacted):

_____

_____

_____

_____

As you prepare to finish with therapy, there will be a number of things you still want to work on. The good news is that you now have the knowledge and skills to do so! This worksheet can help you plan the next steps for each of those goals. Make copies of this worksheet, and use one copy for each goal. Keep them handy so that you can review them regularly.

Decide which goal you want to *continue* working on or *start* working on. Be specific and realistic, and remember that abstract goals and those that are too far out of reach are not as useful.

Goal:

_____

Now that you have a goal in mind, ask yourself the following:

- Is this goal really something *I* want, or is it something *other people* want from me? Make sure the goal is important to *you*.
- Is my standard too high? Can I work on lowering the bar?
- Is this a promotion goal or a prevention goal? If it is a prevention goal (i.e., trying to keep something bad from happening), would I be better off if I focused on *making something good happen*?
- Do I need to learn some new skills to achieve this goal, or do I need to continue improving skills I have already learned?
- How will I be able to tell whether I am making progress on this goal?
- Which worksheets from this book can help me be more effective in working on this goal?

The questions may have prompted you to make some revisions to your goal. After you feel confident that you have a realistic goal, develop a plan for how you will start or continue working on it. Think about what your first steps will be, give yourself a realistic time line, and try to anticipate potential obstacles.

Your Plan:

_____

_____

_____

_____

_____

What obstacles do you anticipate? How will you deal with those obstacles?

_____

_____

_____

_____

_____

Worksheet 26: Being the Person I Want To Be

Make many copies of this worksheet; you will use them every day to help you keep your progress going. **At the start of each day**, write down one behavior (e.g., "getting things done on time") or characteristic (e.g., "being more assertive") that is part of the person you *want to be*. Be realistic and specific.

Write the behavior, characteristic, or goal you will work on today.

Your goal:

_____

List the situations that are likely to happen today that will allow you to practice this behavior, develop this characteristic, or accomplish this goal. How will you remember to follow through with your plan?

Your plan:

_____

_____

_____

_____

At the end of the day:

To what extent did you accomplish what you had planned for today (on a scale from 0 to 5)?

0	1	2	3	4	5

Not at all   Completely

What kinds of obstacles (e.g., practical things, thoughts, feelings, other people) made it difficult for you to carry out your plan today? How could you overcome those obstacles next time?

_____

_____

_____

_____

If you were able to carry out your plan, how did it affect your mood?

_____

_____

_____

_____

Worksheet 27: Challenging Situations

Make many copies of this worksheet; you will use them every day to help keep the progress going. **At the start of each day**, write down one *challenging situation* you will be faced with during that day (e.g., work or school assignment, conversation with a family member).

_____

_____

_____

_____

List your goals for that situation. What do you want to accomplish? What kind of person do you want to be in that situation (e.g., how do you want to behave or handle the situation)? Be realistic.

_____

_____

_____

_____

At the end of the day, complete the following ratings (using a scale from 0 to 5).

How much were you able to accomplish your goals for this challenging situation?

0	1	2	3	4	5

Not at all   Completely

Did your goals for the challenging situation include making something good happen?

0	1	2	3	4	5

Not at all   Completely

Did your goals for the challenging situation include preventing something bad from happening?

0	1	2	3	4	5

Not at all   Completely

What did you learn from this challenging situation that can help you in future situations?

_____

_____

_____

_____

Worksheet 28: Self-Monitoring and Coping After Therapy Ends

The conclusion of this program involves developing a detailed and personal plan to help you monitor your mood and be prepared if you believe it is starting to decline. For the first part of your plan, identify your red flags, which are feelings, physical symptoms, thoughts, or behaviors that serve as warning signs of a decline in mood. Try to think about the *earliest* warning signs you have noticed in the past; they are the most useful ones. For example, some people notice that they do not want to go out of the house as much. Others feel tired all the time even though they have had a good night's sleep.

My Red Flags
1.
2.
3.
4.
5.
6.

Now that you know your red flags, how will you watch out for them? Sometimes, depression has a way of creeping up gradually. Just as a person with diabetes needs to monitor his glucose levels, regular self-checkups are important for people with depression. How will you continue to check in on your mood so that you can spot the warning signs as soon as possible? Enlisting the help of a loved one may be helpful; other people may notice changes that you do not see.

My Mood Check-In Plan
Signs or symptoms I will monitor:
How I will monitor my signs or symptoms (e.g., keeping a log with a rating scale, reviewing my activities from the past week, checking in with a trusted loved one):
How often I will monitor (weekly is ideal, monthly is a minimum):
How I will remember to monitor (e.g., calendar entry, phone alert):

Next, make a coping plan to implement when one of your red flags appears. The coping plan includes things you can do on your own and things that involve other people. On your own, you can use the worksheets and other exercises from this program, increase your physical activity (e.g., taking walks), or do something you enjoy (e.g., watching a favorite movie). Examples of things that involve other people include reaching out to a supportive friend for help, telling your partner about how you are feeling, and making plans with family members.

Things I Can Do to Cope On My Own
1.
2.
3.
4.
5.
6.
7.

Things I Can Do to Cope with the Help of Others
1.
2.
3.
4.
5.
6.
7.

If you have tried all of these things but continue to struggle, it may be time to seek professional help. With the help of your therapist, write down some resources that are available to help you locate an appropriate professional, even if you move to another location.

Resources

Kari M. Eddington, PhD, is a clinical psychologist, Associate Professor of Psychology, and Director of the Depression Treatment and Research Program at the University of North Carolina at Greensboro. She received her PhD in psychology at Indiana University in Bloomington, Indiana, and her research focuses on motivational factors in depression.

Timothy J. Strauman, PhD, is Professor of Psychology and Neuroscience and Professor of Psychiatry and Behavioral Sciences at Duke University. Dr. Strauman is a clinical psychologist who translates behavioral science and brain science research into treatments and preventive interventions for mental disorders. His recent research includes development of self-system therapy; combining psychotherapy and transcranial magnetic stimulation to create more effective treatment options for depression; exploring the emergence of gender differences in depression; and creating a self-regulation model for vulnerability to depression.

Angela Z. Vieth, PhD, is a Visiting Assistant Professor and the Associate Director of Undergraduate Studies for Psychology at Duke University. She earned her MA and PhD in Clinical Psychology from the University of Missouri–Columbia, and completed postdoctoral work at the University of Wisconsin–Madison and Duke University. Her research and teaching interests lie on the border between clinical and social psychology.

Gregory G. Kolden, PhD, is Professor of Psychiatry and Psychology at the University of Wisconsin–Madison, Director of the Psychology Training Program, and Chief Psychologist. Dr. Kolden's research has focused on the evaluation of efficacy of behavioral interventions and the mechanisms underlying the changes that result from these treatments in psychiatric (e.g., mood-disordered outpatients) and medical populations. His work includes meta-analytic examination of psychotherapy relational elements and the use of structural equation modeling to examine the role of nonspecific therapeutic change processes (e.g., aspects of the therapy relationship) in empirically supported treatments.